YOGA

For Busy People

YOGA
For Busy People

BIJOYLAXMI HOTA

Cover Concept, Design & Illustrated By
Praloy Chakravorty

Rupa & Co

Copyright © Bijoylaxmi Hota 2002

First published 2002
Third impression 2004

Published by

Rupa & Co

7/16, Ansari Road, Daryaganj,
New Delhi 110 002

Sales Centres:

Allahabad Bangalore Chandigarh Chennai
Hyderabad Jaipur Kathmandu
Kolkata Ludhiana Mumbai Pune

Printed in India by
Gopsons Papers Ltd.
A-14 Sector 60
Noida 201 301

Thanks to
Dr. P.R. Mishra, Ram Manohar Lohia Hospital
Dr. Srivastava, Ram Manohar Lohia Hospital

Models
Reela Hota   – (cover) Odissi dancer
Manisha   – Chau dancer
Rajat Vohra   – Model

Photography
Harbans Modi (cover)

Layout Artist
Deepa Chakravorty

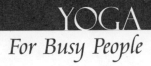

YOGA
For Busy People

Contents

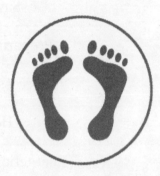

With the blessing of my Guru and Guide
Paramhansa Swami Satyananda Saraswati

Introduction

<u>Yoga — The Saviour</u>

Way back in the 1970s, one night, I suddenly found my fingers twisting and turning. Soon my whole body was convulsing violently. Nothing I did would stop it. I was rushed to the hospital. The doctor examined me, went out of the room and said to his colleague "She has tetany." I heard it as 'tetanus', and to me it sounded no less than a death knell.

Though after an injection, my convulsion subsided, it recurred after a few days. My body was for some reason not absorbing calcium from food. But pathological investigations revealed no abnormality whatsoever. All the milk and calcium tonics which I took were of no use. Convulsions occurred again and yet again. I was told there was no permanent cure for this calcium deficiency related convulsions and only the symptoms could be controlled by a calcium injection. I started fearing the attacks. A casual question of a friend as to what would happen if the muscles of my heart suffered from cramps scared me stiff. Tetany may not be a serious ailment but my reactions were no less than that of a terminally ill patient. I would panic if I was not close to a good hospital. My fear and anxiety led to insomnia which became worse by the day. I was put on tranquillizers. I deteriorated fast, physically and mentally gathering ailments such as acute anaemia, severe backache, cysts

in the uterus, palpitations etc. And then I took to yoga and in two weeks all my problems vanished!

I was wonderstruck by yoga's power and started studying it in depth and later teaching it to help other sufferers. I became busier and busier, travelling and taking 2-4 classes a day. I had no time for my own yoga practice. Punishment was bound to come. Suddenly my stomach stopped functioning. No matter what or how little I ate, it remained in the stomach for the entire day. My weight came down rapidly from 56 kgs to 45 kgs. Again after thorough investigation, the Head of the Department of Gastroentrology of AIIMS announced, "There is nothing wrong with your system. For some reason your inner temperament has changed and we cannot do anything about it". Another death knell!

I started the yogic and dietary treatments, promising myself again and again never to leave it ever in my life. Once again yoga pulled me out of my predicament. I remember I had gone to Australia with a YPO (Young Presidents' Organisation) group to teach yoga in their retreat. At dinner, Tom, a student and a dear friend was watching me piling my plate with sausages, crabs, fish and prawns. He could not believe it when I finished them all. He went and exclaimed to my daughter, "Your mother is crazy, she has actually finished a kilo of meat". I could digest all that only because of my yoga. Touch wood!

As a practitioner of yoga for the last twenty five years and as a yoga therapist for the last twenty years, I have experienced the benefits of yoga on myself and on persons who I have taught. To illustrate, cases of high blood pressure and spondylitis have been controlled within a week to ten days. These patients were on drugs for years before taking up yoga. After yogic treatment, they were off drugs completely. Persons with chronic headaches, with sleep problems, with excess body weight, with diabetes and a host of other ailments have been cured by me through yoga.

A case worth mentioning is of Dr. Vandana, a professor in the U.S. She had a large benign tumour removed in John Hopkins Hospital, Baltimore and was put under medication to prevent any further growth. But when she went for a check-up after three months, a still bigger tumour was found. The doctors expressed their helplessness and admitted that their system had failed and they couldn't do anything more about it. Dr. Vandana came to India for a month and learnt yoga from me. After her return to the U.S. when she went for another check-up there was no tumour! The doctor said that it was nothing but a miracle and that if he did not have the earlier report with him, he would not have believed that she ever had a tumour.

Another case is that of Edith, a Swiss lady who had breast cancer. I suggested certain yogic practices to her which were to be done during the medical tests and treatment she was undergoing. Her body showed no sign of stress during those lengthy and ardous periods nor any reaction of chemotherapy. She never took the maintenance dose for chemo and now after twelve years or so, she is still in the best of her health!

Yoga is a system devised by the ancient yogis of India out of their intuitive knowledge. It has thoroughly understood the mysterious psycho-physiological complex of man.

According to yoga, man is not just flesh, blood and bones but a configuration of a gross body, a subtle energy body, the thinking mind, the psychological mind, the emotional mind and the spirit or soul.

Perfect health is nothing but perfect harmony among all these aspects. Any disharmony anywhere gradually affects all the other parts and the manifestations are seen on the physical body. All problems can be tackled and harmony maintained, by dealing with all the aspects simultaneously, through various yogic techniques.

All these techniques are extremely effective and the effects are felt almost instantenously. Recently I was in Simla for three days in a retreat organised by the Confederation of Indian Industries to teach yoga to its members. On the second day itself a cheerful participant announced in his booming voice, "The high point of this trip is yoga. It is great! Makes me feel so good." Somebody else remarked "but where is the time?" But ailment does not wait for a busy person to become 'un-busy' to attack. Unannounced, it ruthlessly strikes the busiest and makes sure the busy person is made 'un-busy'. It does not spare even the mightiest!

Pope John Paul II, who will be eighty two in May 2002, has the Parkinson's disease. Ronald Reagan, former President of USA, who is a little over eighty years, is in advanced stage of Alzheimer's disease. For the last few years,

Mr. Regan has not been seen in public. The former Chinese President, Deng Ziao Ping, who was responsible for transforming the Chinese economy, was so weak and debilitated because of old age that he was taken care of by a team of trained nurses before his death a few years ago.

One wonders if these famous leaders — a leader of religion and two leaders of powerful countries — would have led healthier lives even in their old age if they had been practising yoga which is believed to prevent all diseases and physical decay due to advancing years.

Yoga is the right remedy for the sick and maladjusted modern society. In the post-industrial modern societies, even school kids commit acts of mindless violence. The act of terrorists crashing airplanes and destroying the twin towers of the World Trade Centre and badly damaging the Pentagon on 11 September 2001 was so ghastly that the world is yet to recover fully from the shock. In a highly industrialised society as in the West, one out of three marriages ends in divorce and one out of three children grows up without a father.

A wise person is he who turns to yoga and maintains perfect physical and mental health all his life and enjoys the fruit of his work better till the very end. As you go through this book, you will realise the various usages of this great science in our lives and how to fit them all in our daily routine.

So, start yoga right away, before it is too late as beyond a point even yoga cannot do much.

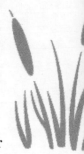

Chapter 2

Flier's Friend

The successful man today is a globe trotting man, flying from one corner of the world to the other. The long hours in an aircraft are not without perils. In recent time, many long distance fliers have met with sudden deaths causing concern the world over.

In the aircraft, a passenger's hands and legs remain inactive. The blood circulation especially the venous return becomes less and less as flying hours become more and more. This diminished venous return causes stasis in the blood vessels which can lead to clot formation. This clot can travel to the heart causing a sudden heart attack.

A simple group of asanas called *Pawanmuktasana* prevents such a calamity by maintaining the optimum health of the blood vessels. Many asanas from this series can be done in the aircraft itself to quickly speed up blood circulation.

Pawanmuktasana

This series puts all the joints into motion and loosens them. By stretching and relaxing the muscles and blood vessels it exercises them properly, making them supple. The stretching movements also squeezes out toxins from the tissues to the bloodstream which are then thrown out of the system by the now healthier eliminative organs.

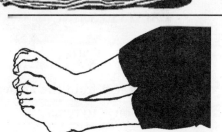

Exercise 1

> Sit on the floor stretching the legs in front.

> Place hands on the floor behind you to support the body.

> Join the feet and keep the toes pointing up.

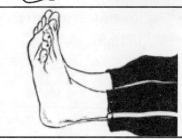

> Bend the toes forward and then backward.

> Repeat 10 times.

Exercise 2

▶ Bend the feet forward from the ankles then bend backward.

▶ Repeat 10 times.

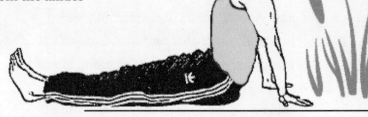

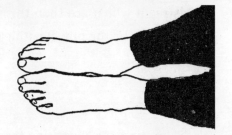

Exercise 3

▶ Move legs apart.

▶ Rotate feet from the ankles in one direction – 10 times.

▶ Rotate feet in the other direction – 10 times.

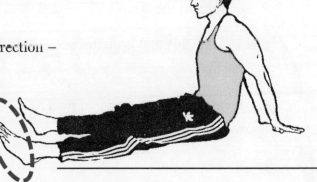

Exercise 4

➤ Place the right foot on the left thigh.

➤ Place the right hand on the right knee.

➤ Hold the right foot in the left hand.

➤ Rotate the right foot with the hand in one direction – 10 times.

➤ Rotate it in the other direction – 10 times.

➤ Repeat it with the other foot.

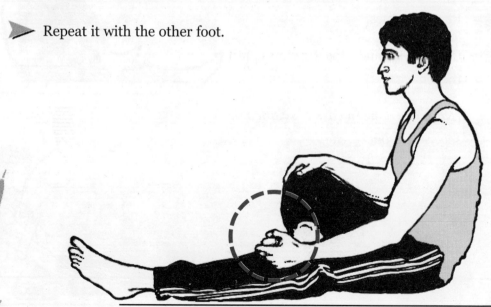

Exercise 5

▶ Stretch legs in front.

▶ Interlock the fingers and hold the right thigh.

▶ Bend the right leg and point the right toe upward.

▶ Straighten the leg and stretch it well with toes pointing out.

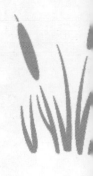

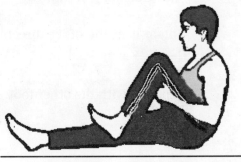

▶ Repeat 7 times.

▶ Change legs and repeat 7 times with the left leg.

(Not to be done in case of sciatica or severe low back-ache)

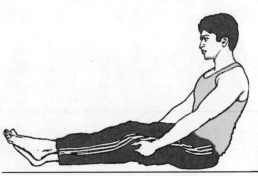

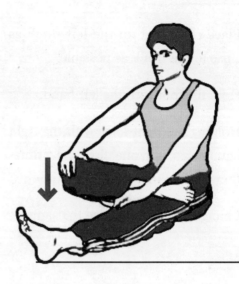

Exercise 6

➤ Place right foot on the left thigh, keeping the left leg straight.

➤ Place hands on the respective knees.

➤ Press the right thigh down towards the floor.

➤ Repeat 7 times.

➤ Change legs and repeat 7 times.

Exercise 7

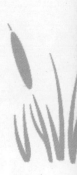

➤ Place right foot on the left thigh as close to the trunk as possible.

➤ Hold the foot with the left hand.

➤ Holding the right knee with the right hand rotate it in one direction 7 times then in the other direction 7 times.

➤ Change legs and practise the same.

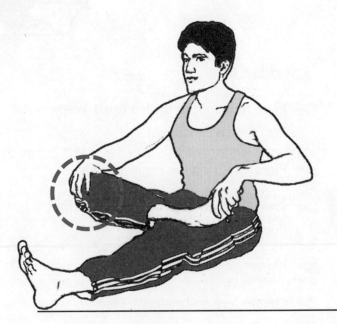

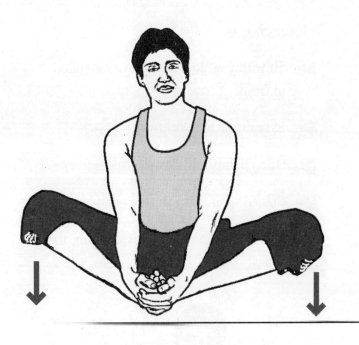

Exercise 8

▶ Bend legs and bring the feet together facing each other.

▶ Hold the feet.

▶ Move knees up and down fast like the flapping of wings 20-30 times.

Exercise 9

➤ Sit with your legs crossed or extended in front.

➤ Extend the arms in front.

➤ Open palms and flex the fingers.

➤ Clench them with thumbs inside.

➤ Repeat clenching and unclenching 10 times.

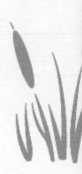

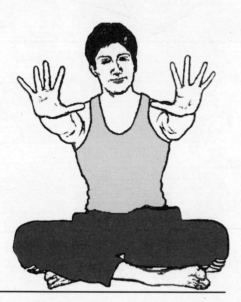 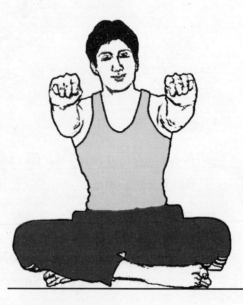

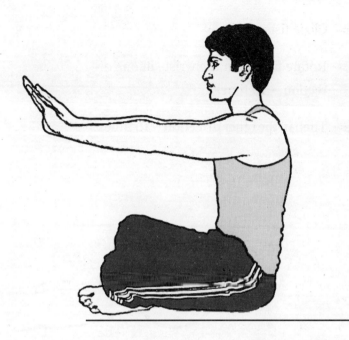

Exercise 10

➤ Join fingers.

➤ Bend hands down from the wrists then upwards.

➤ Repeat 10 times.

Exercise 11

➤ Close fists.

➤ Rotate fists from the wrists in one direction – 10 times.

➤ Then in the other direction – 10 times.

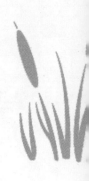

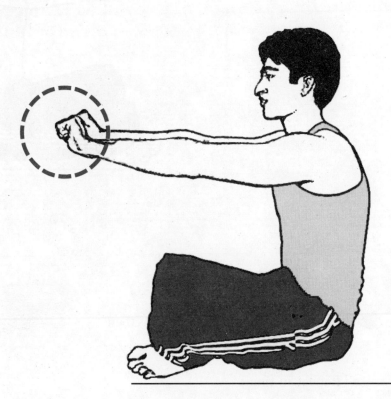

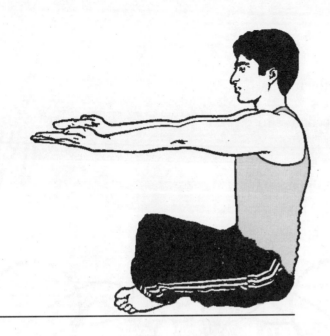

Exercise 12

➤ Join fingers and extend arms in front.

➤ Bend arms from the elbows and touch the shoulders.

➤ Repeat 10 times.

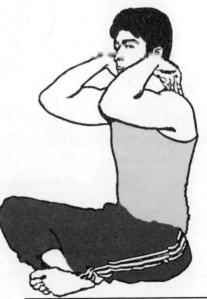

Exercise 13

➤ Touch shoulders with all the fingers.

➤ Rotate elbows in one direction – 10 times.

➤ Then in the other direction – 10 times.

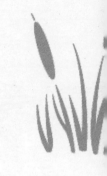

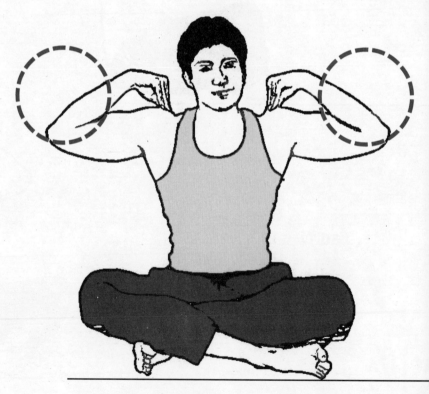

Exercise 14

➤ Keep hands on the lap

➤ Bend head to the left, then to the right.

➤ Repeat 10 times.

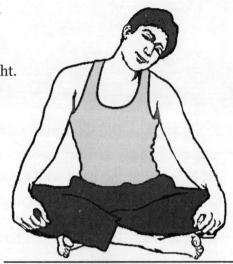

Exercise 15

➤ Turn head to the left then to the right.

➤ Repeat 10 times.

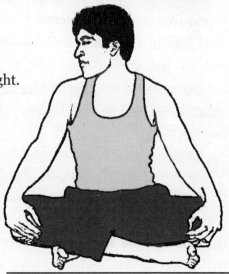

Chapter 3

<u>Save Your Back</u>

Pain in the neck – how true is this cliché! Unpleasant people and situations can actually tense up the neck muscles and cause neck-pain. Continuous bending of the head while working worsens it, resulting in cervical spondilitis which is so common among the busy people of today.

Sitting for long hours on a chair has its own problems. First it causes stiffness and muscle fatigue. Secondly, gravity pulls the vertebrae downwards – especially when the back muscles are unexercised and weak – bringing them close together. The spinal nerves arising from the spinal cord are pressed and the electric impulses moving to and fro from the brain to all body parts are disturbed leading to malfunction of the glands or organs. And when the sciatic nerves are pressed, severe pain at the lower back running down the legs can occur.

Unexercised back muscles can lead to misaligned vertebrae and postural defects resulting in pain and low energy levels.To prevent all such maladies, it is essential to:

(i)   Release the accumulated tension in the back from time to time.

(ii)   Exercise each and every back muscle.

(iii)   Develop correct postural habits.

Asanas to be practised at work place

To release tension from the entire back

and to lift pressure from the spinal nerve,

<u>Tadasana</u>

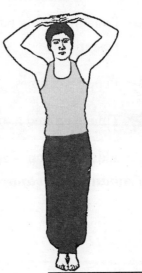

...a natural traction – is very effective. It should be practised 2-3 times during the day.

<u>Technique</u>

➤ Stand with feet close together.

➤ Interlock fingers and keep hands on the head.

➤ Inhaling, raise hands above the head and stand on the toes.

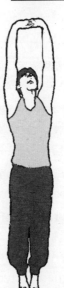

➤ Look up and stretch well.

➤ Hold the posture for as long as you can hold your breath.

➤ Exhaling, come back to the starting posture.

➤ Repeat 5-7 times.

➤ Time – around 2 minutes.

Shoulder rotation – Exercise No. 13 of *Pawanmuktasana*

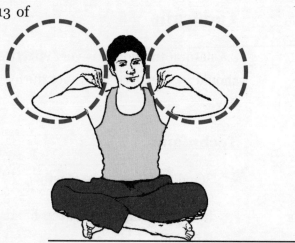

Asana to be practised at home to strengthen the back.

<u>Bhujangasana</u>

This 'asana' relaxes the back muscles, strengthens the back and relocates misaligned vertebrae.

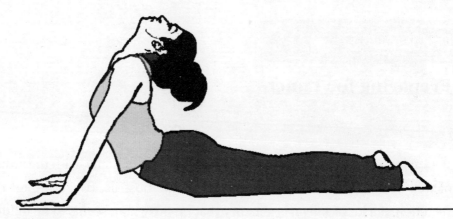

Technique

- Lie down on your stomach, face down.

- Place palms on the floor beside the chest.

- Inhaling, slowly raise the trunk with face turned up.

- The abdomen should remain on the floor.

- Hold the posture for one or two seconds.

- Exhaling, lower yourself.

- Repeat 3 times.

Gradually increase the duration to hold the posture for as long as you can hold the breath.

Increase the number to 5.

Chapter 4

Preparing for Lunch

Having a meal leisurely, in the cosy atmosphere of home, with the aroma of well cooked favourite dishes drifting to the nostrils, triggering off the secretion of a lot of saliva, is a luxury that no busy man seems to be indulging in today's world.

Lunch has now become a hurried affair, taken at the workplace with a mind agitated or preoccupied with various problems.

Behaviour of the stomach was studied thoroughly by studying a patient recovering from a healed gunshot wound. It was observed that every time the man was stressed, the stomach shed its lining and became raw. Taking food under such a condition can only lead to ill health.

Relaxing before meals is quickly achieved by the following practice.

➤ Sit comfortably and close your eyes.

➤ Breathe naturally.

➤ Count breaths backward from 27.

➤ Relive a funfilled event of your life or remember a beautiful place.

➤ Visualise yourself having a hearty meal and feeling empty in the stomach soon after.

➤ Open your eyes.

Before you have your meal also check the flow of breath in the nostrils. We usually breathe from one nostril at a time, the flow changing at specific intervals. According to Yoga, the right nostril is connected with the left hemisphere of the brain which controls the physical actions of the body including digestion and the left nostril breathing indicates heightened mental action and diminished physical action. Taking food at such time can cause

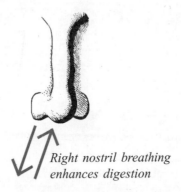

Right nostril breathing enhances digestion

impaired digestion. Eat while the right nostril is active. If the left is flowing, it can be changed by the following practice, though it is better to wait till it changes naturally. (In people with health problems the rhythm is highly disturbed which can be corrected through appropriate yogic practices).

Technique

Press armpits with opposite hands leaving the thumb out for 2-3 minutes. Remove the left hand and check the flow. If it has not changed repeat it again.

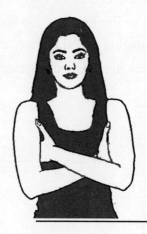

After the meal if possible sit in ***Vajrasana*** for 10 minutes to ensure smooth digestion. In this asana blood is pooled near the stomach giving it extra energy to work better.

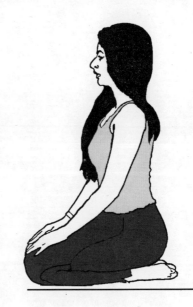

Technique

- Kneel down, feet joined.

- Sit on the heels.

- Place hands on the legs.

To still enhance digestion, imagine a whirlpool of golden light rotating behind the navel or concentrate on the energy center 'Manipura Chakra' corresponding the solar nerve plexus. In yoga, Manipura Chakra is the controlling center of digestion. Looking at a picture of this chakra also helps.

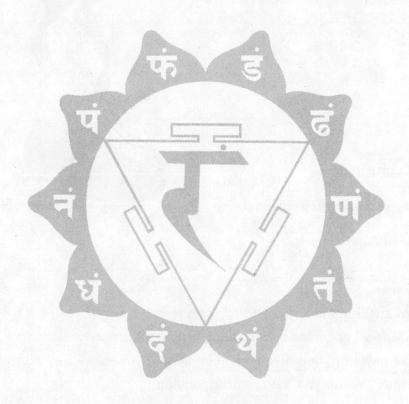

Manipura Chakra

Chapter 5

Success in Meetings

Meetings are a part of a working man's daily routine. Deals are clinched, differences are sorted out, policies are formulated and problems are solved. It does not pay to become stressed before or during an important meeting. A tense mind is a handicap – it is inefficient and inaccurate.

An examinee may forget various vital points in the examination hall, but as soon as he leaves it, the information comes flooding back. Information come better from a highly relaxed mind.

Also a relaxed person can influence others positively and get their co-operation, which an agitated person can never achieve. Agitation spreads around and repels people. Nervousness too is counterproductive. Not only does it project a weak and unattractive image, it leads to various physical discomforts such as palpitation, dry mouth and a churning stomach.

To overcome all such undesirable symptoms, and to relax quickly, certain yogic techniques are extremely useful. The techniques can be practised anywhere and in any position but to learn them properly, it is essential to follow the prescribed method.

Abdominal Breathing

(also improves brain functions by providing it with extra oxygen)

➤ Assume Shavasana (lie down on the back with feet one-and-a-half feet apart).

➤ Place hands away from the body with the palms turned upward.

➤ Close eyes and relax.

➤ Inhale slowly filling up the lower part of the lungs first, so that the abdomen rises.

➤ Inhale further to fill up the upper part of the lungs so that the chest rises next.

➤ Inhale still more and let the shoulder move up.

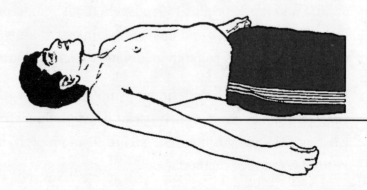

➤ Now the entire lungs are full.

➤ Hold the breath for a few moments.

➤ Exhale to release the air first from the chest and then from the abdomen.

➤ Practise it for five minutes.

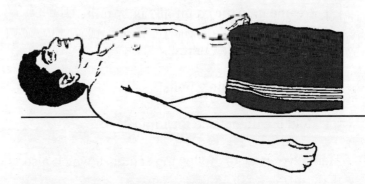

☐ It seems difficult in the beginning but with regular practice it becomessmooth and wave-like.

☐ To further enhance the effect, mentally repeat "I am inhaling peace" as you inhale and "I am releasing anger" as you exhale.

Use of Mantra to control palpitation

☐ Use any short mantra such as Om, Amen, Amin, Rama, Allah or Jesus.

☐ Inhale slow and deep breath, repeating the mantra mentally.

Hold the breath for a second. Exhale slower still repeating the mantra at the same speed but double the number of mantras during inhalation. Like if you repeat the mantra five times while inhaling, repeat it ten times while exhaling, so that the ratio of inhalation and exhalation is 1:2.

To over come nervousness

☐ Breathe in to the count of 7 i.e. 7 units.

☐ Hold breath for 1 unit.

☐ Breathe out again 7 units.

☐ Hold breath outside for 1 unit.

Mentally repeat the following sentence which also is divided into 7 units, both during inhalation and exhalation.

For example : O   God   make me   calm and   composed.

(1   2   3   4   5   6   7)

Use the interim unit to count the number of rounds backward.

For example :

- While inhaling say "O God make me calm and composed"

- Hold breath and say – "Twenty Seven"

- While exhaling say again "O God make me calm and composed"

- Hold breath and say –"Twenty Seven"

- In the next round it is "Twenty Six" instead of "Twenty Seven"

- Count from 27 to 1.

Note : An atheist can substitute his or her own name for God. For example a Rajesh can say,"O Rajesh Please Be Calm And Composed."

Chapter 6

Health Booster

Physical exercise is necessary to remain healthy but never overexercise! As with medicine, an underdose is useless and an overdose can kill, so also with physical exercise. It is only the right dose that does the trick. Asanas or yogic postures have been around for millennia proving their safety and efficacy in maintaining perfect health of its practitioner.

Asanas are the mainstay of **Hatha Yoga** – the yoga of the body. They are often likened to physical exercises which they are not. In fact they are diagonally opposite to each other in their function and effects.

In physical exercise, the oxygen consumption goes up.
During asanas it is conserved – more oxygen means more strength and energy through oxidation of glucose in the body.
Secondly, exercises give rise to hard muscles.
Asanas make them supple – elasticity spells better health than rigidity.
Thirdly, exercises increase the bulk of the muscles. Large muscles use up much more oxygen and also strain the heart which has to supply blood to all those extra muscle cells.

Asanas do not increase the bulk beyond the healthy limits.

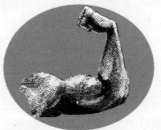

Large muscles use up more oxygen

It must be kept in mind that a heavy man may not be able to break a brick with one hand, but a child can do so with an expert karate chop.

Strength and vigour come not from bulky muscles, but from the amount of energy in the body. Higher the energy level, healthier we feel. This energy in yoga is called *prana*. Prana is the vital life force that keeps a man alive. More the prana in the body, more alive the person is. And when it leaves the body, the person dies – even though the composition of the body remains unchanged.

Prana is bioplasmic energy, said to be finer than atomic energy. It was known to mankind since antiquity. It is called *rauch* in Hebrew, *ki* in Japan, *chi* in China, and *manna* in Hawai. Science has now captured it in photographs and measured its voltage with sophisticated instruments.

According to yoga, prana is absorbed into the body from the atmosphere and then stored in the chakras or energy centers which also distribute it throughout the body. There are myriad chakras in the body and the six most important of them are located on the spine corresponding the nerve plexi.

Various factors can make the chakras sluggish leading to energy depletion and ill health. Asanas were designed to activate them and maintain their optimum health.

Scientific research on the effects of asanas shows —

1. increased blood flow to the brain and other vital organs

2. healthy stimulation of the brain tissues

3. increased blood flow to the organs while they remained relaxed.

Suryanamaskar

Of all the asanas Suryanamaskar is a complete technique suiting most busy people of today. It is a group of asanas devised to tone up all the systems of the body. It is dynamic, slimming and highly invigorating.

Note: People with a weak back or high blood-pressure should not attempt this practice.

Pose 1

Stand with feet joined and hands folded in front of the chest.

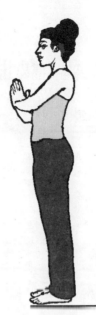

Pose 2

Raise hands and bend backward.

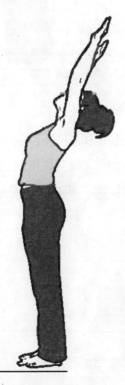

Pose 3

Bend forward and place the hands flat on the floor. You may bend the knees in the beginning.

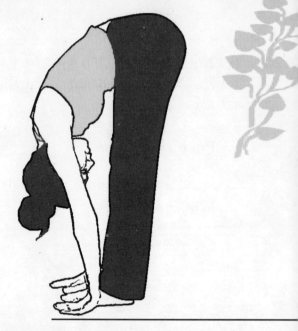

Pose 4

Stretch the right leg back while bending the left knee & lowering the torso. Stretch the neck backwards.

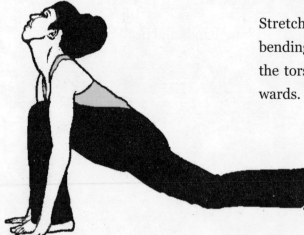

Pose 5

Lifting the hips take the left foot back to join the right foot. Lower your head. The body assumes a triangular position.

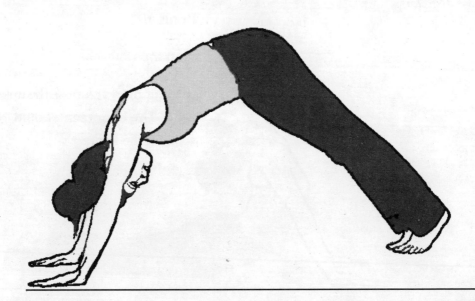

Pose 6

Lower the body to the floor. Let the chin, chest and knees rest on the floor but not the stomach.

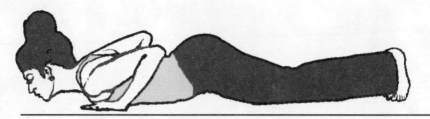

Pose 7

Drop the stomach.

Lift your head and raise the upper body. The abdomen should remain on the floor.

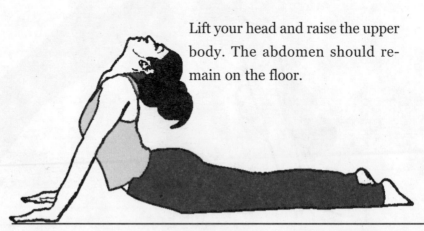

Pose 8

Lift the hips up to the triangular
position of pose 5.

Pose 9

Bring the left foot forward and
assume pose 4.

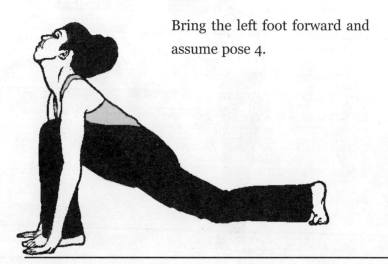

47

Pose 10

Straighten your legs and raise hips as in Pose 3.

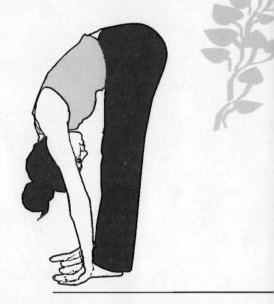

Pose 11

Raise hands above your head and bend backwards.

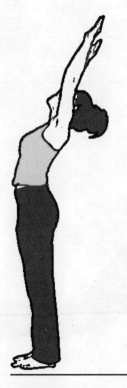

Pose 12

Fold hands and bring them down to the chest, like in the starting position.

To complete one round, one such cycle has to be done with the right foot in front and left leg stretched back.

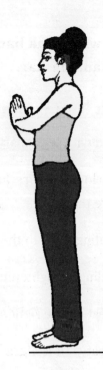

Breathing

Inhale while assuming	pose 2
Exhale while assuming	pose 3
Inhale while assuming	pose 4
Exhale while assuming	pose 5
Hold breath while assuming	pose 6
Inhale while assuming	pose 7
Exhale while assuming	pose 8
Inhale while assuming	pose 9
Exhale while assuming	pose 10
Inhale while assuming	pose 11
Exhale while assuming	pose 12

People with weak back should do the following 4 asanas instead of Suryanamaskar.

<u>Triyak Tadasana</u>

➤ Stand with legs apart.

➤ Interlock fingers and raise hands above the head.

➤ Exhaling bend to the left.

➤ Inhaling straighten up.

➤ Repeat on the right side.

➤ Repeat 7 times, gradually increasing the number till you reach 10 rounds.

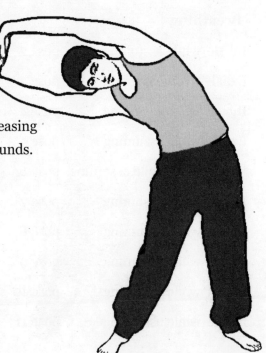

Kati Chakrasana I

- Stand with feet apart.

- Extend arms in front.

- Swing to the left from the waist.

- Swing to the right.

- Repeat 7 times, gradually working up to 15 times.

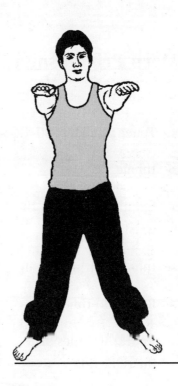

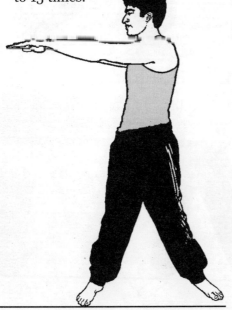

Meru Prishtasana

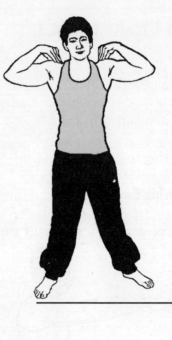

> Stand with feet apart.

> Touch shoulder with respective hands.

> Inhale.

> Exhaling bend to the left from the waist.

> Inhaling straighten up.

> Repeat 10 times.

> Repeat 10 times on the right side.

Kati Chakrasana II

➤ Stand with feet apart.

➤ Extend arms to the sides.

➤ Swing to the left from the waist moving the arms to place the right hand on the left shoulder and the left hand on the right side waist.

➤ The left palm should be turned out.

➤ Swing to the right side and change the hands.

➤ Repeat 7 times, gradually increasing the number to 10.

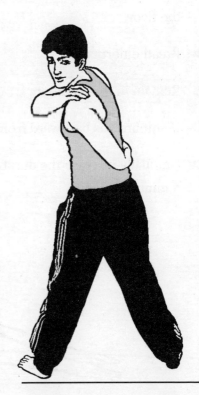

Shashankasana

> Sit in Vajrasana.

> Inhaling raise hands above the head.

> Exhaling bend forward.

> Place the forehead and forearms on the floor.

> Breathe normally.

> Remain in that position.

> Count breaths backward from 10 to 1.

> Gradually increase the duration to 2-3 minutes.

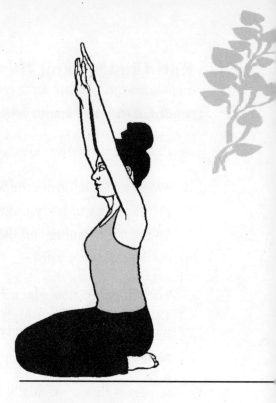

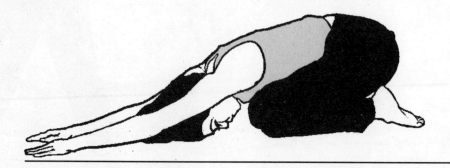

Note: *It is important to rest the forehead on the ground and not let it remain suspended. If the body is stiff, you may place a cushion on the heels and sit on it.*

To normalise an overactive adrenal gland and control anger, shashankasana is the most effective. People with uncontrollable temper can practise it for as long as half an hour.

Shavasana

➤ Lie down on your back in a straight line.

➤ Move legs one-and-a-half feet apart.

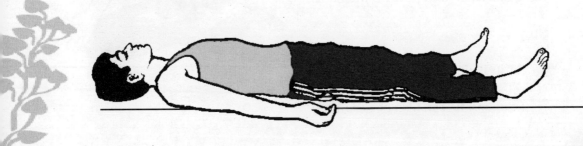

- Place hands on the floor (palms facing up), away from the body.

- Close eyes.

- Breathe naturally.

- Count 10 breaths backwards.

    Shavasana relaxes the body in the shortest time.

Nadisodhan Pranayama

Energy in the body flows through energy pathways called *nadis*. Excessive thinking and over excitement often creates blockages in these energy pathways obstructing its free flow. Nadisodhan pranayama is a breathing technique that removes these blockages and purifies the nadis.

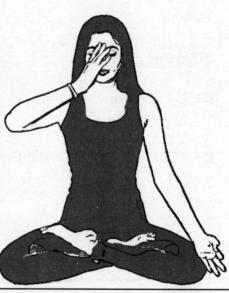

Step 1

- Sit in Padmasana i.e. lotus pose.

    (Sukhasana can also be assumed)

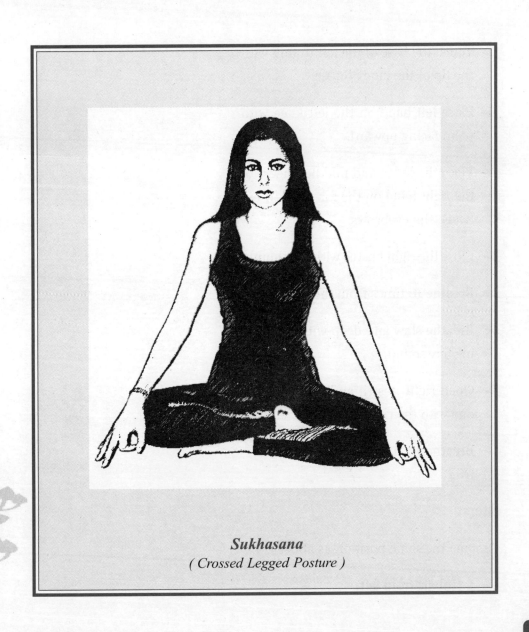

Sukhasana
(Crossed Legged Posture)

- Touch the base of the left thumb with the tip of the index finger.

- Place left hand on the left knee with palm facing upward.

- Place the index and middle fingers of the right hand on the forehead in between the eyebrows.

- Close the right nostril with the thumb.

- Breathe 10 times from the left nostril.

- Breathe slow and deep without making any sound.

- Open right nostril and close the left one with the ring finger.

- Breathe 10 times from the right nostril.

Step 2

Assume the same position as above.

- Inhale from left.

- Close left nostril with the ring finger.

- Open the right nostril and exhale.

- Close right nostril with the thumb & open the left one.

- Repeat 10 times. Repeat on the other side.

Step 3

Practise in the same manner but alternate the nostril i.e. inhale from left, exhale from right and inhale from right, exhale from left.

- Repeat 10 times.

Step 4

- Assume the same positure as above. Inhale from left.

- At the end of inhalation close both nostrils and retain breath inside.

- Open the right nostril and exhale.

- Inhale from the same (right) nostril.

- Close both nostrils retaining the breath.

- Exhale from the left.

- The ratio of inhalation, retention and exhalation should be 1:1:1.

- Repeat 10 times.

Chapter 7

Energetic in the Evenings

After a busy day, invariably a man heads for the bar. No harm. In the vedas *somras* – an intoxicating drink — occupied a very high place. Many verses are dedicated to its praise. Devotees of Lord Shiva regularly take an intoxicating drink – *bhang*. The virtues of intoxicants are well described in an interesting story about Birbal.

Once, in Emperor Akbar's court a man jealous of Birbal's popularity wanted to poison the Emperor's mind by informing him that Birbal was a habitual drunkard. Akbar was enraged but he wanted to find out the truth for himself. So in the evening, he went to Birbal's house and hiding himself well, peeped in. Lo and behold, Birbal poured himself a drink, looked at it and said, "This one is for my health" and drank it. He poured another drink and looking at it said, "This one is for beauty". He drank that too. Then he poured the third drink, looked at it and said, "This one is poison for me" and threw it away.

Alcohol may make you feel nice and high, but never in excess. Oxygenation of the system after a day's mental work is more effective to banish tiredness.

Mental work, especially in a stressful situation, leads to shallow breathing which uses the upper part of the lungs only. This results in inadequate oxygen intake and building up of carbon dioxide, making one feel tired and lethargic. To oxygenate the system it is necessary to first expel the stale air from the lungs and then breathe well using the whole lung, which is done best by the following yogic techniques so that the blood is thoroughly oxygenated and one feels fresh and rejuvenated.

Agnisar Kriya

- Sit in Vajrasana.

- Move knees apart.

- Place hands on the knees.

- Drop chin to the chest.

- Lift the shoulder.

- Stick tongue out.

- Pant like a dog.

- Repeat 20 times.

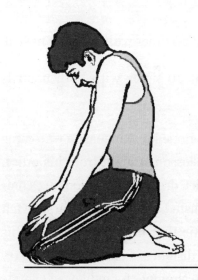

<u>Kapalbhati Pranayama</u>

➤ Sit with legs crossed.

➤ Place the first and second fingers of the right hand on the forehead in between the eyebrows. Place the left hand on the left knee with the index finger touching the base of the thumb. Close right nostril with the right thumb. Breathe 20 times rapidly from the left.

➤ Inhale automatically but exhale with a force.

➤ Repeat 20 times with the right nostril.

➤ Repeat 20 times with both nostrils open.

I remember one Mr. Ringenson who came for a yoga lesson straight from his office, his shoulder drooping, and looking complete exhausted. But after the class, he felt so energetic that he walked back to his house — a distance of about 10 k.m. So try the above techniques for enhanced energy.

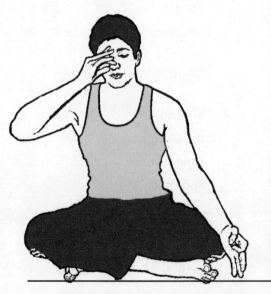

Chapter 8

The Great De-stresser

Many an ordinary man has demonstrated unimaginable strength and speed in the face of danger - be it fighting fire or fleeing from a tiger. It is possible only due to the stress mechanism of the body that provides it with the extra energy it needs during an emergency. But to get back the lost energy, the body needs to be completely rested and de-stressed.

For the busy man of today, stress has turned from a boon to a bane. The continuous stress of his daily life creates more problems than one can imagine. Not only do all ailments spring from it but it also ruins one's efficiency, relationships and peace of mind.

We cannot wish away the stress factors as there are too many of them ranging from noise to traffic jams to unpleasant neighbours. It is also not possible to release stress by just wanting to. One needs a technique to do that and meditation is the proven technique.

Thousands of meditative techniques have been developed the world over to suit different people as no two people are alike in their needs, capacity and mental make-up. Though all of them have the same effects on the body and mind, mantra meditation popularly known as transcendental meditation or TM suits the modern busy man the most because of its simplicity and relaxed rules.

Studies in the West show that during mantra meditation –

(ii)   heartbeat slows down

(iii)   blood-pressure falls

(iv)   oxygen consumption is reduced

(v)   lactate, a stress hormone is eliminated four times faster from the body than during sleep

(vi)   the brain produces strong alpha waves – all indications of heightened relaxation and reduced tension.

Another research finding suggests that a practioner of meditation may have an increased ability to express his feelings freely and a reduced level of anxiety. Also, many practioners of TM have reported finding it easier to give up the use of various habit-forming drugs including marijuana, amphetamines and barbiturates.

The highly de-stressed condition of the meditator also leads to stability in the nervous system and glandular system. As the endocrine system controls not only all physical functions of our body, but also our emotions, meditation improves our emotional and psychological well-being too.

Mantra meditation is one practice that does not require the meditator to sit in a meditative pose or to close the eyes, making it easy for the stiff bodied restless modern man. Also, it can be practised anywhere. A busy man with time constraint can even do it in the car while returning home from work provided he is not driving himself. All he needs is to go on repeating the mantra either mentally, audibly or just whisper for twenty-thirty minutes – the time required to bring about the necessary positive changes in the system.

If you do not have a guru to choose a mantra for you, use any mantra that catches your fancy. Mantras are of three types –

1) Religious
2) Psychic and
3) Universal.

Stay clear of psychic mantras. They may prove too powerful for you to handle. All religious and universal mantras are absolutely safe. Once practised for a while the mantra should not be changed. Mantra is a vibratory mystic energy which permeates each corner of the person's body and mind and a new mantra might create disharmony in the personality.

Using a mala or rosary is optional though many gurus insist on it.

Rudraksh is the most favoured mala as it suits all mantras. For certain religious mantras, specific malas are used. For example: Crystal is used for Devi Mantra and basil for Vishnu Mantra.

Technique

Relax. Try not to move the body during the practice and repeat the mantra. Maintain your awareness of the mantra. But if the mind wanders do not force it back, just follow it. After a while gently bring it to the mantra again.

Some Mantras

Religious

❏ Om Namah Shivaya

❏ Hari Om

❏ Amen

❏ Amin

❏ Arhint

❏ Vahe Guru

❏ Asham Vohu

☐ Om Manipadma Hum

Universal

☐ Om

☐ Soham (I am that)

☐ Aham Brahmasmi (I am consciousness)

☐ Tat Twam Asi (You are that)

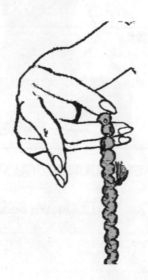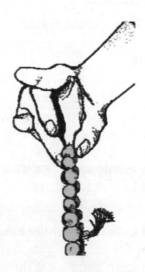

Correct ways of holding the mala

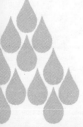

Psychic Mantras

- Hreem

- Haum

- Dum

- Aim

Om Meditation

(a powerfull anti-depressant)

Technique

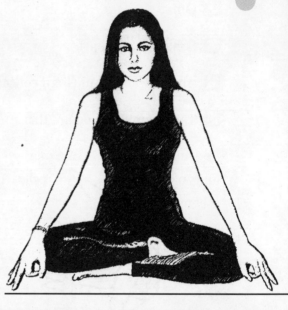

- Sit in a meditative pose.

- Take a deep breath.

- As you exhale say - OOOOOOOOOOOO UUUUUUUUUUUU MMMMMMMM

- At the same time go on repeating ...Om Om Om (1 Om per Second)
  till you have emptied the lungs.

- Inhale again and repeat the same process.

- Practise it for 10 to 15 minute twice daily.

Chapter 9

<u>Yogic Sleep</u>

Perhaps the high point of yoga and the most enjoyable of all its techniques is *yoganidra* or yogic sleep. Its effect is to be experienced to be believed. It relaxes the body as nothing else does.

The muscular tension of a man's body when measured by EMG showed 37 units of tension while he is reclining on an easy chair, and 20 units when he is lying on the bed. This shows that whether we are sitting or lying or doing any physical work or not, we still have some physical tension. The tension normally leaves the body when a man has a sound restful sleep. Such sleep is also required to repair the daily wear and tear of the body.

But man rarely gets natural sound sleep. His mind continues to think, plan and worry throughout the day. At night, even after the person falls asleep, due to the day's worries he usually has a poor and disturbed sleep. By the morning, the body is only half rested, and half repaired, and he goes on accumulating physical and mental tension all through the day. Like the tighter and tighter winding of a clock spring, the body too becomes more and more tense leading to many tension-related ailments and speedy degeneration of the body's tissues which in turn results in premature old age and related debilitating conditions.

Deep relaxation and sound sleep are essential to check the rapid degeneration of body tissues and their regeneration. This can be easily attained by yoganidra. It is a practice developed from an ancient tantric practice by my guru Paramahamsa Swamy Satyananda Saraswati. It systematically and thoroughly relaxes each part of the body and induces deep sleep. Wherever I have conducted yoganidra, by the end of the ten minutes, majority of the participants would be asleep — some of them even snoring.

Research on yoganidra has revealed many wonderful results.

First the brain waves during yoganidra become predominantly alpha. It indicates a state which psychology calls hypnogogic, and is considered as the most restorative state. It also indicates a highly alert mental state with sharpened intellectual abilities. People have used this state to learn new languages in an amazingly short time. The subconscious mind becomes more receptive during yoganidra, and any suggestion made to it in such a condition always succeeds. People have used this technique to

(i)   give up a harmful habit

(ii)   acquire a beneficial one

(iii)   re-programme the mind

(iv)   achieve skill

(v)   attain success

(vi)   reduce physical pain considerably

According to psychologists, there are natural mechanisms in the spinal cord that sometimes close, preventing messages of pain from reaching the brain. Brain can direct this gate from the spine to close or open as it wants. During deep relaxation induced by yoganidra, the brain usually transmits messages to close the gate and thus messages of pain do not reach the brain and pain is not felt.

Yoganidra should be practised every night before sleep to unwind the day's tension and to induce better sleep. It has been seen that half-an-hour of yogic sleep gives the same benefit as two hours of deep sleep. Such a sleep, no doubt, is ideal to rejuvenate the entire body and mind.

Yoganidra can also be practised during the day provided the stomach is not full. Leave a gap of at least two hours after a meal to practise it.

Though yoganidra can be practised in any position, shavasana is thought to be the best for its practice.

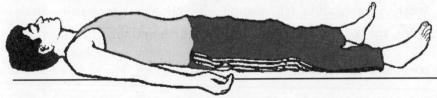

*** 30 minutes of yoganidra is equal to 2 hours of deep sleep.**

Technique

Lie down in shavasana

Take 12 deep breaths while mentally saying —

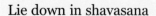 "I am inhaling – Twelve"

 "I am exhaling – Twelve"

 "I am inhaling – Eleven"

 "I am exhaling – Eleven"

 Till you reach – 1

Now breathe naturally and repeat mentally 'relax' after each exhalation.

Practise for three-four minutes.

Visualise each part of the body in the following sequence. Mentally repeat its name and imagine it relaxing. Do not move the said body part. "Right hand thumb - index finger - middle finger - ring finger - little finger - palm - wrist - elbow - shoulder - armpit - hip - thigh - knee - calf - ankle - heel - sole - the big toe - second - third - fourth and the fifth."

Repeat with the left side.

"Back - back of the head - top of the head - forehead - right eyebrow - left eyebrow - right eye - left eye - middle of the eyebrows - right cheek - left cheek - right nostril - left nostril - upper lip - lower lip - chin - neck - chest - stomach and abdomen."

Now make a resolution

Use a short positive sentence, such as –

"I will attain and maintain perfect health."

Or

"I am perfectly healthy in body and mind."

You can use any other sentence and repeat it every day.

Imagine you are standing near a waterfall and capture every detail about the area – sight, sound and smell. It should be a highly pleasant and relaxing experience.

If you are not particularly fond of waterfalls, imagine a sea beach or a calm lake.

Visualise the following healing symbols.

Starlit night, full moon, rising sun, setting sun, pink lotus, blue lotus, white lotus, wisp of a white cloud, blue sky and candle flame.

Repeat your resolution again 3 times again.

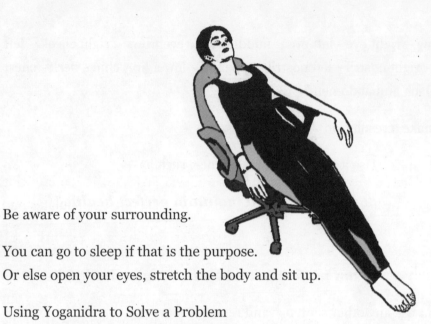

Be aware of your surrounding.

You can go to sleep if that is the purpose.
Or else open your eyes, stretch the body and sit up.

Using Yoganidra to Solve a Problem

i)   At night practise yoganidra.

ii)   When you are about to sleep, tell the problem to your subconscious mind and ask for a solution.

iii) The all-knowing and all-powerful subconscious mind will solve it at night and present the solution to you in the morning.

iv)   Sometimes it may require a few more sessions to workout the solution but when it does you will be amazed at its efficiency.

(Yoganidra can be recorded in an audio cassette and listened to for better relaxation)

Chapter 10

System Cleansers

Stress and faulty food habits slow down the movement of the intestine leading to insufficient evacuation of the bowel. The filth accumulates and rots in the colon and soon becomes the breeding ground for germs, bacteria and parasites which produce toxins that find their way to the various body parts through the blood stream. The skin that receives such dirty blood is bound to look dull and starved; and the glands and organs that are fed with this poisonous blood become weak and ineffective. Furthermore, the cells irritated by the toxins can go haywire and multiply fast causing perhaps tumors and cancer.

The Royal Society of Medicine, London has announced that almost every chronic disease is directly or indirectly due to bacterial poisons absorbed from the intestine. No wonder diseases are on the rise. It is said that two out of every five people living today will have cancer.

Laghoo Shankh Prakshyalan is an excellent yogic technique to cure constipation.

This technique should be done in the morning before taking anything at all, tea included.

Note :
Elderly people must consult their physicians before taking up this practice.

☐ Take six glasses of warm water.

☐ Add one level tsp. salt (can be more or less according to requirement).

☐ Drink two glasses quickly.

☐ Practise the following five asanas.

Tadasana

It is the same tadasana described earlier, but here you don't hold the posture for long and in this bring the heels forcefully down, banging the floor with them. So, raise heels, stretch and down with a thud. Repeat 8 times.

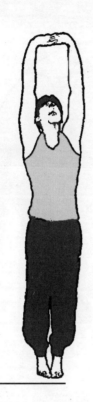

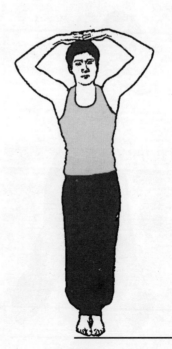

Triyaka Tadasana

Already described.

Repeat 4 times.

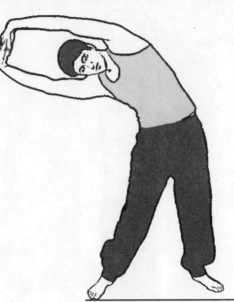

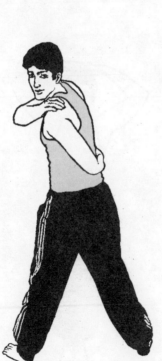

Kati chakrasana – II.

Already described.

Repeat 4 rounds.

Triyak Bhujangasana

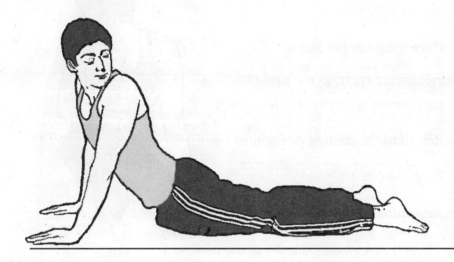

➤ Lie down on the floor, face down.

➤ Place hands beside the chest.

➤ Inhaling rise, turning to the left look
at the feet.

➤ Exhaling go down.

➤ Repeat on the right side.

➤ Repeat four times.

Udarakh

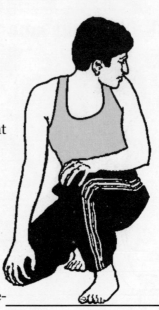

- Squat on the floor.

- Place hands on the knees.

- Twisting the body to the left place right knee on the floor near the left foot.

- Return to the starting position.

- Repeat on the right side.

- Repeat four rounds.

Most people cannot do Udarakh in the beginning. They can instead do the following:

- Sit on a chair.

- Lifting bended legs up, grasp them under the knees.

- Pressing the legs against the abdomen move them from side to side.

This movement will massage the lower abdomen.

Repeat the entire process twice and visit

the toilet.

- ☐ Do not rest until you feel like visiting toilet.

- ☐ You may have one or two motions.

- ☐ It may be a little watery too.

- ☐ If you don't see any change in that, next time add ½ tsp more salt.

- ☐ And if it is too watery or you pass stool too many times, reduce the salt by ½ tsp.

- ☐ Food should be taken after an hour when you feel hungry.

Laghoo Shankha Prakshyalan should be done fortnightly for a clean system.

Note: People with high blood pressure must not do this Kriya.

Kunjal and Vyaghrakriya

Kunjal and *Vyaghrakriya* are one and the same i.e. induced vomiting. The only difference is that Kunjal is done on an empty stomach in the morning while Vyaghrakriya is performed anytime to remove the food from the stomach. Kunjal strenghens the digestive organs and Vyaghrakriya saves the system from offending or poisonous food. Unless extremely uncomfortable, wait for 4 fours after the food is taken to do Vyaghrakriya.

Technique

☐ Add 1 ½ level tsp of salt in 6 glasses of warm water.

☐ Drink from it as much as you can and as fast as possible.

☐ Immediately throw up by inserting two fingers in the mouth and touching the throat to induce wretching.

☐ The water will come out gushing.

☐ Continue till no water comes.

☐ Add only 1 tsp of salt the first time you try this technique. If you succeed in throwing up, you can increase the amount. Do not strain to vomit. If it does not happen, try next week.

☐ Food must not be taken for at least 30 minutes after completion of kunjal.

☐ Vyaghrakriya leaves the gullet sore and burning due to the excessive stomach acid. To soothe that take milk and rice gruel sweetened with honey.

Neti

(To clear the nasal passage for better oxygenation of the system)

☐ Fill up a neti vessel with warm (a little higher than body temperature) and saline (same as your tear) water.

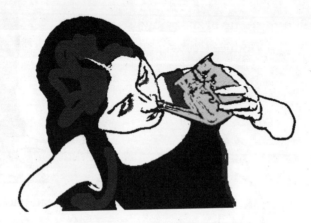

☐ While breathing through the mouth pour water from one nostril to the other and out.

☐ Repeat from the other nostril.

☐ Blow nose gently.

☐ Remove water by remaining in the following posture for 30 seconds each, still breathing from the mouth.

(i) Bend forward

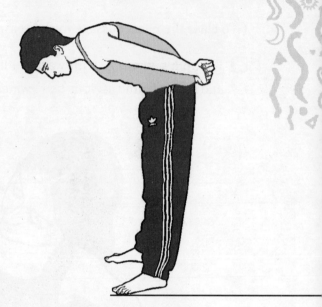

(ii) Bend head backward

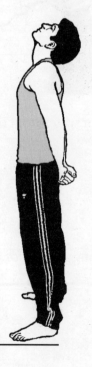

(iii) Lie face down on the stomach

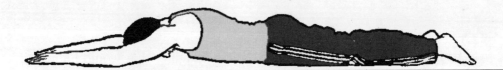

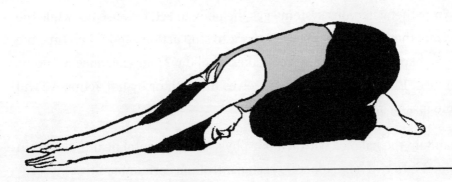

(iv) Shashankasana

If all the water is not drained out repeat the postures once more.
Dry up the nostrils (important) by *Kapalbhati pranayama*.

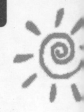

Chapter 11

Complimentary Activities

The universe exists because of a balance. Imagine what would happen if the balance is tipped? There will be complete chaos leading to dissolution.

We exist because of such balances — balance between the north pole and south pole; between physical and mental energies and between the sympathetic and parasympathetic nervous systems.

The sympathetic nervous system eggs the body to act, to tense up, while the parasympathetic nervous system urges it to stop actions and relax. Imagine what can happen when one system takes a holiday? Our existence would be threatened. Either we will work ourselves to death or by not acting we will become insane and waste away.

To maintain the balance between our physical and mental health, the brain is divided into two hemispheres, each controlling certain faculties. According to yoga the busy man of today mostly uses the left hemisphere, which controls calculation, comparison, planning and logical thinking. He needs to consciously include certain activities that will force his right brain to function.

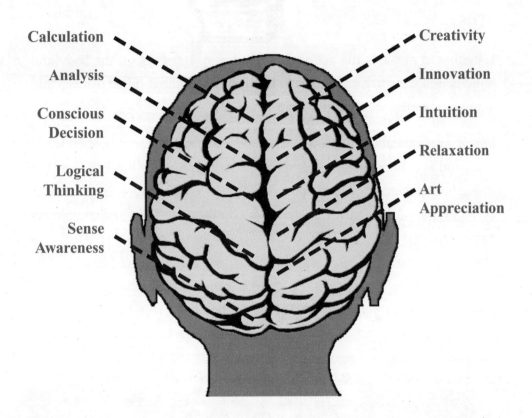

Calculation

Analysis

Conscious
Decision

Logical
Thinking

Sense
Awareness

Creativity

Innovation

Intuition

Relaxation

Art
Appreciation

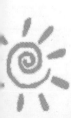

Some of them are as follows-

<u>Music</u>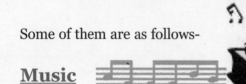

Listening to music is the act of the right brain. Its effect on the body and mind is well known. A baby even in its mother's womb is lulled to sleep and a milch cow increases its milk yield.

Music automatically pulls man's attention like a magnet and holds it while the mind is calmed and the nerves are soothed. Studies have shown that music boosts memory. Elderly people with background music have remembered events of their past in details which otherwise they had completely forgotten.

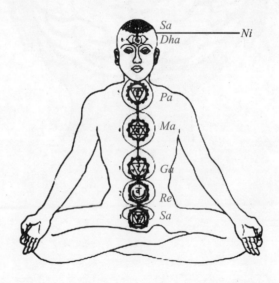

Accordingly to yoga, the seven notes of music correspond to the seven major chakras on the spine. The tunes produce a resonance on the chakras setting them into correct motion.

Studies also have revealed that steady regular rhythm for thirty-forty minutes helps release stress.

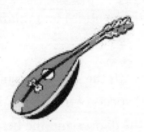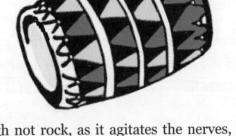

Therefore, listen to music, though not rock, as it agitates the nerves, but soft classical ones. And try to participate in it by drumming hands against an object, tapping the foot or simply by clapping.

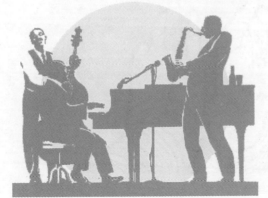

De-stressing

Dance

The fluid graceful movements of dance are extremely pleasing to the eyes and mind. The artful and precise twisting, turning and bending activate the myriad chakras present all over the body. Combined with music and rhythm it becomes all the more effective. Indian classical dance still has an edge over other dance forms as it imbibes *bhakti* (devotion) and *mudra* (hand gestures) too.

Mudras belong to hathayoga and they play with the energy circuits of the body in a positive manner. And by depicting aspects of the Divine, it tries to generate love and devotion in the minds of the dancer and the beholder.

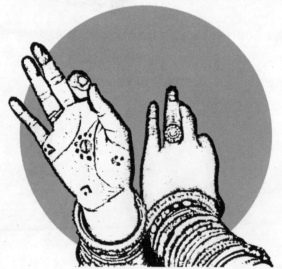

Mudra (Hand gesture) affects the energy within

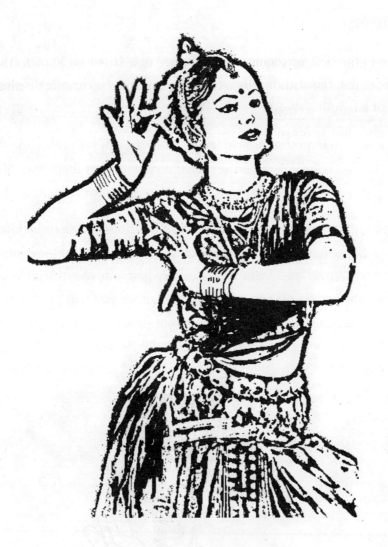

Indian Clssical Dance

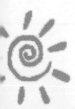

Laughter

Laughter is the best medicine — so say the wise. In a well known book by the same name, the author tells us how he cured his incurable disease by a bellyful of laughter a day.

People now have forgotten how to laugh. They are always preoccupied with their problems. It is high time they tried a dose of this medicine. Many a cardiologists prescribe ten minutes a day of laughter for a healthier heart.

One can have a natural laugh by watching a hilarious movie or by joining a group practising *hasya yoga* (yoga of laughter). Since laughter is most infectious it will surely make you laugh; or else just induce artificial laughter. By moving the same muscles in the same manner you will be able to trick the brain to release the same chemicals that produce positive reactions in the body. People view funny and distorted reflections of themselves on special mirrors to induce laughter. Choose anything, do any trick, but guffaw!

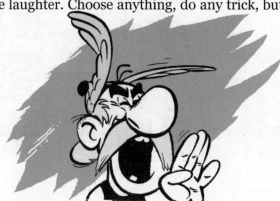

Painting

This too is a right brain activity. When you choose to paint for health reasons, a little knowledge of the effects of colours on the body and mind is helpful.

Red – Stimulates digestive fire, increases energy, encourages extroversion and aggression and counters depression.

Orange – Improves elimination, induces optimism.

Yellow – Improves digestion, strengthens nervous system and creates cheerfulness.

Green – Soothes the nerves and tones up the heart.

Blue – Cools the body, calms the mind and induces sleep.

Indigo – Strengthens the nerves especially of the eyes, counters negativity of the mind.

Violet – A mystic colour that stirs spirituality.

Chapter 12

Advice and Instructions

Moderation Mantra : Fitness Freak – what an apt term for the modern, educated man who gurgles down gallons of water and gorges on salads. For him something good means more of it is better. How wrong! Studies have revealed the harmful effects of anything taken in excess, as can be seen in the following passages.

Water is the elixir of life: blood, hormones and digestive juices are made from it; toxins from body are removed through it; and plumpness of the skin is retained because of it.

But excess water washes away sodium from body tissues. As sodium is essential to maintain the osmotic pressure in the cells, with its depletion, the cells lose their fluid and get dehydrated. Salt deficiency also causes muscular cramps and low blood pressure. If left untreated this can result in a life-threatening situation — hyponatraemia. Water also dilutes and washes away other minerals from the cells. In extreme cases, due to excessive intake of water, electrolyte balance of body fluid alters, leading to collapse of the lungs or a heart attack.

Excessive intake of water increases workload of the kidneys. Kidney specialists think even eight large glasses of water per day for a normal person

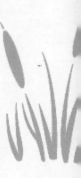

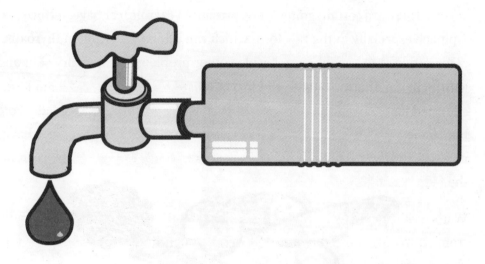

More than 800 chemicals are found in potable water

can be considered as excessive. Some highly eminent urologists have come to the finding that an average-sized adult with healthy kidneys, and living in a temperate climate needs no more than one litre of fluid per day.

With too much intake of water, body's exposure to pollutants also increases. More than 800 chemicals including pesticides and insecticides have been found in good quality potable water. Nitrates may also be present in potable water which can react with other chemicals to form potentially carcinogenic compounds. Another dangerous chemical in potable water could be traces of aluminium, which is linked with the dreaded Alzhmeimer's disease.

Salad – The slimmers diet! But fresh salad taken in excess can backfire on them! There are certain goiterogens present in carrots, cabbage, lettuce and spinach especially in the raw form which can inhibit secretion of thyroxine. This can lead to weight gain, besides other problems such as dry skin and brittle hair, lethargy, fatigue and forgetfulness.

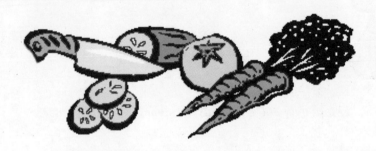

High Protein Diet – Also favoured by slimmers and of course by sportspersons. It can increase uric acid in the body which stiffens joints causing very painful diseases as arthritis and gout.

Soyabean – Though a healthy alternative to animal protein, too much of it can inhibit absorption disturbing function of the thyroids and the resultant disturbances in bodily functions.

Vitamins – Too much of

1) Vitamin C inhibits absorption of copper leading to degeneration of brain tissues.
2) Vitamin A causes hair loss, dry skin, joint pain and even liver damage. During pregnancy, excess intake of Vitamin A can even cause birth defects.
3) Niacin can aggravate diabetes and damage the liver.
4) Vitamin B6 or pyridoxine can cause irreversible nerve damage.
5) Vitamin E - the wonder antioxidant which also is said to preserve youth and vitality can lead to fatigue, nausea and diarrhoea.

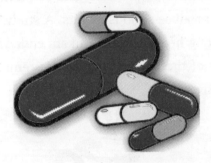

<u>Minerals</u> – Calcium taken in excess can stiffen muscles and joints making movement painful in old-age.

Too much zinc in food or drink shrinks blood cells and impairs immunity against disease.

Food Items – Excessive intake of cereals leads to obesity, cardiovascular degeneration, hardening of liver and defective metabolism. It has been established that nutmeg taken in excess excites the mortor cortex and can produce epileptic convulsions. It can also cause lesions in the liver. Poppy seeds taken in excess can cause renal calculi, so does excessive lime.

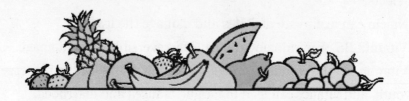

Coffee – Too much coffee causes high acidity and palpitation of the heart. During pregnancy, it can produce serious results. A study showed that 13 out of 16 pregnancies among heavy coffee drinkers ended in spontaneous abortion or stillbirth; out of the balance two were premature births and only one was a normal delivery.

Cola – The caffeine present in cola drinks decreases the absorption of iron and removes calcium from the system, leading to anaemia and osteoporosis. Children who are highly sensitive to caffeine tend to become hyperactive if they drink too many bottles of cola.

Tea – Excessive drinking of tea increases fluoride in the body which damages the teeth and bones including the spinal column. Over a period of excessive intake of tea, the spine loses its flexibility resulting in severe pain.

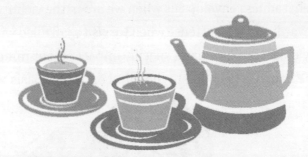

Exercise – Studies have shown that overexercising the body decreases the number of white blood cells leading to impaired immunity against diseases.

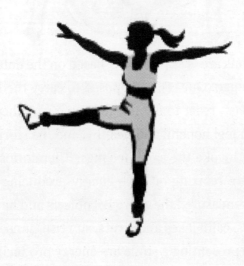

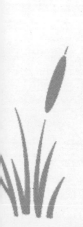

Meditation– Even excessive meditation lowers the inner temperature which is so important for digestion and in the long run can be very harmful.

Objects of Desire – Sombre feelings flood us in a temple, mosque or church; sadness envelops us when we are in the vicinity of a burning ghat or graveyard; and we feel tense when we visit a jail filled with killers and dacoits. Every object or place has a specific impact on our mind and we cannot help it. The data has been fed to the mind on whose basis we react.

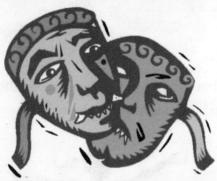

Many of our reactions are very primitive, based on the data fed to the primitive man millennia ago. Our cells, supposed to carry the history of our entire evolutionary past, react to stimuli the same way they reacted then. If the sun made them feel hopeful and healthy, and the storm caused them to tense up, they still invoke the same feelings. Therefore surround yourself with objects that are relaxing or have energy producing qualities. People have indigeneously measured the energy of objects and have found that pictures of gods, saints, calm lakes and rivers, sun rise, sunset, smiling people, even half a circle representing a smile are energy producing.

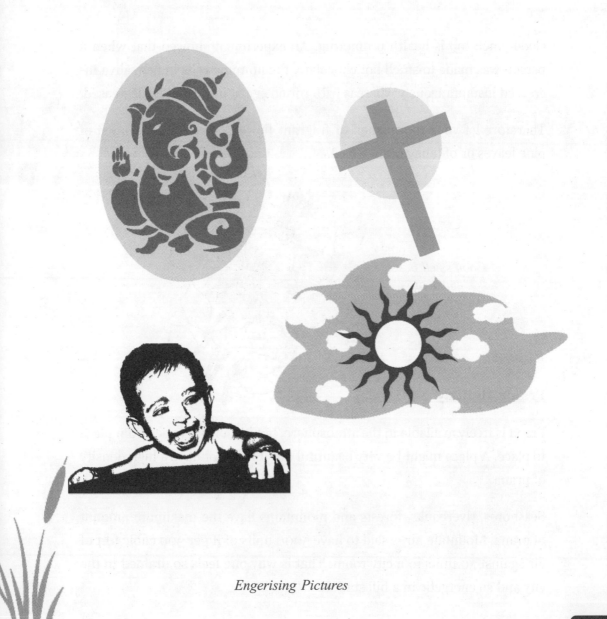

Engerising Pictures

Good smell too is health promoting. An experiment showed that when a person was made to smell hot chocolate, the immune cells in her saliva increased instantaneously whereas with rotten egg, it immediately decreased.

Therefore let your room smell of fragrant flowers, or the crispy smell of pine leaves or of tangy orange peel.

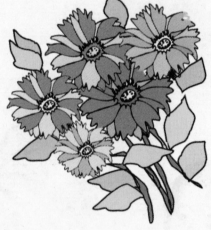

Good smell boosts immunity

Pranic Holiday

Prana is freely available in the atmosphere, but its density varies from place to place. A place might be very beautiful but it may not have a high density of prana.

Seashores, riverbanks, forests and mountains have the maximum amount of prana. Mountain air is said to have 5000 units of it per 300 cubic feet of air against 50 units in a city room. That is why one feels so drained in the city and so energetic in a hill station.

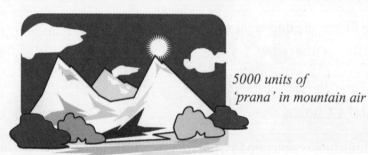

5000 units of 'prana' in mountain air

Therefore, get away to the mountains whenever possible, even for a day or two and practise pranayama and abdominal breathing as much as you can. All the stored acidic gases of your tissues will be out of your system replenishing it with clean fresh pranic air – instant rejuvenation!

Most Avoidable

Negative thoughts – It has been seen that negative thoughts run through the system and cause the release of neuropeptides which oxidise LDL, a component of cholesterol. This form of LDL cholesterol is sticky which results in cholesterol deposition in the blood vessels narrowing them, a dangerous condition, that can result in a heart attack.

Even saying 'no' has many unpleasant effects on the body. It has been observed that this word causes a physical withdrawal. The glandular, muscular and nervous systems tighten themselves to a condition of rejection while the word 'yes' alters the situation pushing the systems forward.

Studies have shown that gossiping and back biting too have the same reactions on the system as negative thoughts.

So follow the universal golden rule – See no evil, hear no evil and speak no evil. Otherwise you will harm nobody but yourself.

Right Choice

Think before you pop in a pill for every little discomfort. No allopathic medicine is without its harmful side-effects. Medicines are chemicals which pollute and poison the system, sapping energy and vitality, beside causing various other problems. Here are a few examples of the harmful after-effects of modern allopathic medicine to change the attitude of some to take a pill for every ill.

Pain killers are highly habit forming. The body gets used to a dosage after a while, so that the dosage has to be increased from time to time. Secondly, they suppress the body's natural pain-fighting mechanism making the person more intolerant to pain leading to more intake of painkiller – a vicious cycle. Thirdly, regular use of painkillers causes inflammation of the tender stomach lining and causes great damage to digestion.

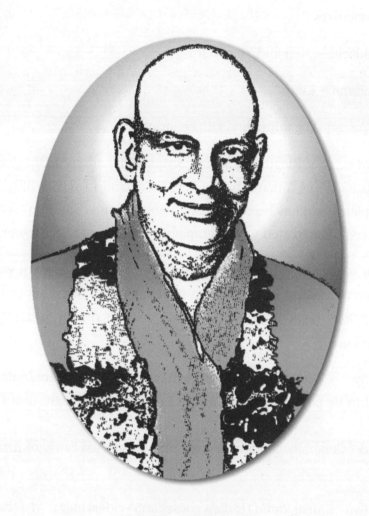

The great saint of Rishikesh...
Swami Sivananda

- [ ] Alternatives

- [ ] Headache – Neti and Yoganidra

- [ ] Migraine – Kunjal

- [ ] All pains – Yoganidra and Om chanting.

The great saint of Rishikesh, Swami Sivananda, had used Om chanting in hospitals including a maternity center in England to successfully alleviate pain of patients. It has been seen that highly painful conditions such as arthritis need to be treated with therapeutic yoga for an effective cure.

Aspirin – After an exhaustive study of a few thousand cases, it was found by a team of medical researchers in the United Kingdom that even a low-dose but long-term aspirin therapy carries the risk of gastrointestinal haemorrhage.

Alternative – Clove, nutmeg (just a pinch) and mace, which are Indian spices, are said to be powerful blood-thinners and can be substitutes of aspirin.

Antacid - Generally contains aluminium - suspected cause of Alzheimer's disease.

Alternative - Kunjal, *amla* (Indian gooseberry) cidervinegar - (1 tbs vinegar + 1 tbs honey in 1/2 cup hot water before meals)

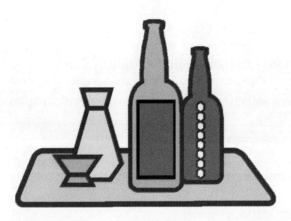

Anti-hypertensive drugs – They can suppress the secretion of the hormone testosterone leading to impotency. Their long use also slows down peristalsis of the intestine leading to gas and constipation which are the root cause of many other diseases.

Alternative – Yoga can normalise high blood-pressure within a week or ten days.

Sleeping pills – The REM factor (Rapid Eye Movement stage) which is vital to rest and rejuvenation of the body is absent in sleep induced by sleeping pills.

Alternative – Yoganidra.

Antibiotics – They destroy the intestinal flora, the organisms so vital to synthesise vitamin B complex, leading to its deficiency and resulting in indigestion and acute debilitating condition.

Alternatives

· Urinary infection – Laghoo Shankha Prakshyalan

· Digestive system infection – Laghoo Shankha Prakshyalan

· Respiratory system infection – Kunjal & Neti

Boost up the immune system with yoga.

Nasal decongestants

Long use can attrophy the nasal lining causing the loss of the sense of smell.

· Alternative – Neti

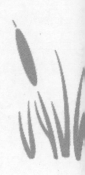

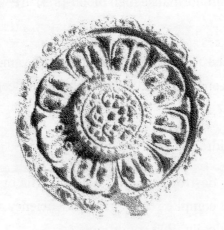

Rules of Yoga

1. All yogic practices should be practised on an empty stomach.

2. Face east while practising yoga. You can also face north for meditation.

3. Do not practise yoga during fever.

4. If you do not get positive results in 3-4 weeks, stop the yogic practices and consult an expert. You may be doing it incorrectly.

5. Do not force your body beyond its limits. Regularity and gentle prodding will win it.

6. Though traditionally yoga is practised early in the morning as the atmosphere is charged with prana then, it can be practised anytime during the day or evening.

7. Wear loose clothes to enable the skin to breathe.

8. Practise yoga in semidarkness and in a well ventilated room.

9. Ladies should not practise yogic 'asanas' in the first four days of monthly period. Meditation and yoganidra can be practised.

Chapter 13

<u>Learning Yoga Step by Step</u>

1st day

Pawanmuktasana

Shavasana – 10 breaths

Nadisodhan Pranayama (Step I)

2nd day

Pawanmuktasana

Shavasana

Tadasana

Triyak Tadasana

Katichakrasana II

Shavasana

Nadisodhan Pranayama

3rd day

Pawanmuktasana

Shavasana

Tadasana

Triyak Tadasana

Katichakrasana I

Meruprishtasana

Katichakrasana II

Shavasana

Agnisar Kriya

Shavasana

Nadisodhan Pranayama

4th day

Pawanmuktasana

Shavasana

Suryanamaskara

Shavasana

Nadisodhan Pranayama

5th day

Suryanamaskara

Shavasana

Bhujangasana

Shashankasana

Shavasana

Nadishodhan Pranayama (Step II)

6th day

Pawanmuktasana

Shavasana

Triyaktadasana

Katichakrasana – I

Meruprishtasana

Katichakrasana – II

Shavasana

Bhujangasana

Shashankasana

Shavasana

Nadisodhan Pranayama

Kapalbhati Pranayama

7th day

Suryanamaskara

Shavasana

Bhujangasana

Shashankasana

Shavasana

Abdominal breathing

Nadisodhan pranayama (Step III)

The Complete Programme

<u>Time</u>

Pawanmuktasana - 5 minutes

Shavasana - ½ minute

Suryanamaskar - 7 minutes

And/Or

Triyak Tadasana

Kati Chakrasana - 7 minutes

Meru Prishtasana

Kati Chakrasana

Shavasana - 2 minutes

Bhujang - 3 minutes

Shavasana - ½ minute

Shashankasana - 3 minutes

Shavasana - 1 minute

Nadisodhan pranayama (Step IV) - 3 minutes

25 minutes

The programme can be divided into two parts to be alternated.

(a)

Pawanmuktasana - 5 minutes

Shavasana - ½ minutes

Bhujang - 3 minutes

Shavasana - ½ minutes

Shashank - 3 minutes

Shavasana - ½ minutes

Nadisodhan Pranayama - 3 minutes

15½ minutes

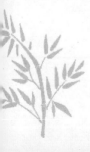

(b)

SuryanamaskarA

Or

Standing asanas - 7 minutes

Shavasana - 2 mintues

Shashank - 3 minutes

Shavasana - ½ minutes

Nadisodhan pranayam - 3 minutes

Total time: 15½ minutes

If some days you have only 7-8 minutes to spare, practise

Pawanmuktasana - 5 minutes

Shavasana - ½ minutes

Nadisodhan Pranayam - 3 minutes

On week-ends clean the system by doing laghoo shankh prakshalan and kunjal one day and kunjal and neti on the other day. For laghoo shankh praksyalan salt should be added on alternate days, i.e. one Sunday add salt and next Sunday add no salt in the water.

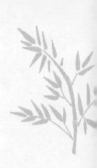

Though 10 to 30 rounds of Suryanamaskara are generally practised, one can practise it as many times as one wants.

More asanas can also be added if desired.

People with high blood-pressure should normalise their B.P. before practising agnisar kriya, kapalbhati pranayam and any yogic practice which involves breath retention.

Yoga should be practised at least thrice a week (alternate days) to get any benefit. Nothing like practising it everyday. Remember – nothing comes easy in life – money, fame, power or even good health. One has to exert for it.

Perseverance always pays !

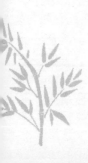

References

1. Eat to Heal – Kristine M. Napier - Warna Books.

2. Be your own Doctor - Ann Wigmore – Every Publisher Group.

3. Nutrients A to Z - Dr. Michael Sharon, Rupa & Co.

4. Medicinal Secrets of your Food – Dr. Aman.

5. I am Joe's Body – J.D. Ratcliff Berkley Books, New York.

6. Mayo Clinic Family Health Book Publisher William Morrow & Company, Inc. New York.

7. Introduction to Psychology – Ernest R. Hilgard, Rita L. Atkinson and Richard C. Atkinson, Harcourt Brace Jovanorich Inc.

8. Psychology 3rd Ed. – Robert A. Baron Prentice Hall of India Pvt. Ltd., New Delhi.

9. The Silva Mind Control Method – Jose Silva and Philip Miele, Pocket Books.

10. The Silva Mind Control Method For Getting Help From Your Other Side - Jose Silva with Robert B Stone, Pocket Books

11. Health and Hygiene - Swami Sivananda, Divine Life Society

12. Japa Yoga - Swami Sivananda, Divine Life Society

13. Mind - Its Mysteries and Control - Swami Sivananda, Divine Life Society

14. Sure Ways for Success in Life & God Realization - Swami Sivananda, Divine Life Society

15. Concentration and Meditation - Swami Sivananda, Divine Life Society

16. Hatha Yoga - Yogi Ramacharaka, D.B. Taraporelala Sons & Co. Pvt. Ltd.

17. Fourteen Lessons in Yogi Philosophy and Oriental Occultism, D.B. Taraporelala Sons & Co. Pvt. Ltd.

18. Autobiography of a Yogi - Paramahamsa Yogananda

19. Hatha Yoga Pradipika - Bihar School of Yoga, Munger

20. Asana Pranayam Mudra Bandh - Swami Satyananda Saraswati, Bihar School of Yoga

21. Yoga Nidra   - do –

22. Meditation from Tantra   - do –

23. Self Realisation   - do –

24. Yogic Cure for common diseases   - do –

25. Teachings of Swami Satyananda Saraswati – Vol. I, IV, & V Bihar School of Yoga.

26. Meditation and mantras   - Vishnu Devananda.

26. The ancient science & art of Pranic healing – Choa Kok Sui Pub – Health Accessories For All.

Index